A Guide to
STI's and STD's
for Teens and Young Adults

Comprehensive Information on Sexually Transmitted Diseases and Infections

Kayleigh Lee

Contents

Introduction

This book is more than just a resource; it's a tool for empowerment.

It's an invitation to young individuals to take charge of their health, understand the risks associated with sexual activities, and learn how to protect themselves and others.

It's a stepping stone towards a future where informed choices lead to healthier lives.

STI VS STD

Is there a difference?

The terms "Sexually Transmitted Infection" (STI) and "Sexually Transmitted Disease" (STD) are often used interchangeably, but they have distinct meanings:

Sexually Transmitted Infection (STI)

Definition: An STI is the presence of an infection in the body that is transmitted through sexual contact. This includes a wide range of viruses, bacteria, parasites, and fungi that can be passed from one person to another during sexual activity.

Symptom Status: STIs often do not show any symptoms. Many people can have an STI without knowing it because they do not display any signs of illness.

Focus on Infection Stage: The term STI emphasizes the infection stage of the illness. It recognizes that a person can be infected without having the disease, i.e., they can carry and transmit the infection without having any signs of the disease.

Sexually Transmitted Disease (STD)

Definition: An STD refers to the diseases that result from an STI. It is the advanced stage of an STI, where the infection has caused a significant medical condition or illness.

Symptom Status: STDs are characterized by symptoms. When an STI progresses into a disease, it typically shows symptoms or signs that can be clinically diagnosed.

Focus on Disease Stage: The term STD is used when an STI has developed into a more serious disease state, leading to health problems or symptoms that are clinically recognizable.

Reasons for Preference of STI Over STD

Early Detection and Prevention: Using the term STI highlights the importance of early detection and treatment, even when symptoms are not present.

Reducing Stigma: The term STI is also seen as less stigmatizing than STD. Since many people with STIs do not have symptoms and are not diseased, the term STI can be less judgmental and more accurate.

In many contexts, STI and STD are used interchangeably, but it's important to understand the distinction between an infection (which might not show symptoms) and a disease (which presents clinical symptoms).

Both terms underscore the importance of preventive measures, early detection, and appropriate treatment to manage and control these infections and diseases.

Bacterial STIs

Chlamydia

(Caused by Chlamydia trachomatis)

Chlamydia is a common sexually transmitted infection (STI) caused by the bacterium Chlamydia trachomatis. It can infect both men and women and can cause serious, permanent damage to a woman's reproductive system.

Understanding Chlamydia

Chlamydia is an infection caused by the bacterium Chlamydia trachomatis. It is most commonly transmitted through sexual contact with an infected person. The infection can affect several areas of the body, including the genitals, eyes, and respiratory tract, but most commonly affects the cervix and urethra.

How is it Transmitted?

Chlamydia is primarily transmitted through:

- Vaginal, anal, or oral sex with someone who has the infection.
- Sharing sex toys that have not been washed or covered with a new condom each time they are used.
- It can also be passed from a pregnant woman to her baby during childbirth.

Symptoms in Women

- Abnormal vaginal discharge
- Burning sensation when urinating
- Pain during sexual intercourse
- Bleeding between periods or after sex
- Abdominal pain

Symptoms in Men

- Discharge from the penis
- Burning sensation when urinating
- Pain and swelling in one or both testicles (less common)

Other Symptoms

- Rectal pain, discharge, or bleeding
- Conjunctivitis (if exposed in the eyes)
- Throat infection (if exposed through oral sex)

It's important to note that many people with Chlamydia may not experience any symptoms. This is why regular screenings are crucial, especially for sexually active individuals.

Diagnosis of Chlamydia

Nucleic acid amplification tests (NAATs): The most accurate tests for diagnosing Chlamydia.
Urine tests: Can detect the presence of the bacterium.

Swab tests: Taking samples from the cervix, urethra, rectum, or throat.

Treatment for Chlamydia

Chlamydia is usually treated with antibiotics such as:

- Azithromycin
- Doxycycline

Other antibiotics may be used for those allergic to these medications.

Follow-Up

It's important to abstain from sexual intercourse until the treatment is completed and the infection is fully cleared.

A follow-up test may be recommended several weeks after completing treatment to ensure the infection has been eradicated.

Prevention of Chlamydia

- Using condoms correctly every time you have sex.
- Limiting the number of sexual partners.
- Regular STI screenings, especially if you have multiple sexual partners.

Education and Awareness

Being informed about STIs and their transmission. Open communication with sexual partners about STIs and STI testing.

Chlamydia, although a common and potentially serious STI, is treatable and preventable. Regular screenings, safe sex practices, and timely treatment are key to managing and preventing this infection.

If you suspect you might have Chlamydia, or if you are sexually active, regular check-ups and open discussions with healthcare providers are essential for maintaining good sexual health.

Gonorrhea

(Caused by Neisseria gonorrhoeae)

Guide to Gonorrhea (Caused by Neisseria gonorrhoeae) Gonorrhea is a sexually transmitted infection (STI) caused by the bacterium Neisseria gonorrhoeae. It's known for its quick transmission and potential to cause severe complications if left untreated.

Understanding Gonorrhea

Gonorrhea is a bacterial infection that is easily spread and affects primarily the genital tract. The bacteria can also grow in the mouth, throat, eyes, and anus.

Transmission

Gonorrhea is transmitted through sexual contact with the penis, vagina, mouth, or anus of an infected partner. It can also be spread from mother to baby during childbirth.

Symptoms In Women

- Increased vaginal discharge
- Painful urination
- Vaginal bleeding between periods
- Pelvic pain

Symptoms In Men

- Painful urination
- Pus-like discharge from the penis
- Swelling and pain in one or both testicles (less common)

Other Symptoms

- Rectal pain, discharge, and bleeding
- Conjunctivitis (if the eyes are affected)
- Sore throat (if the throat is affected)

Many people with gonorrhea do not have symptoms, especially women. When symptoms do appear, they are often mild and can be mistaken for a bladder or vaginal infection.

Diagnosis of Gonorrhea

Nucleic Acid Amplification Tests (NAATs): Highly sensitive tests that can identify gonorrhea bacteria. Swab Test: Samples taken from the affected area (throat, urethra, cervix, or rectum) for analysis.

Treatment for Gonorrhea

Effective treatment for gonorrhea usually involves the use of antibiotics such as ceftriaxone and azithromycin. It's crucial to complete the entire course of prescribed antibiotics even if symptoms disappear.

Resistance Concerns

Gonorrhea has been showing increasing resistance to certain antibiotics, making it crucial to use the correct treatment and follow-up to ensure the infection is completely cleared.

Partner Notification and Treatment

Sexual partners should be informed, tested, and treated if necessary, to prevent the spread of the infection and reinfection.

Prevention of Gonorrhea

- Consistent and correct use of condoms during sexual activity.
- Limiting the number of sexual partners.
- Mutual monogamy with a partner who has tested negative for STIs.

Regular Screening

Regular screening is important, especially for sexually active individuals, to detect and treat gonorrhea early.

Avoiding Douching

Women should avoid douching as it can increase the risk of developing a gonorrhea infection.

Gonorrhea is a common STI that requires prompt attention and treatment. With effective treatment, gonorrhea can be cured without lasting effects. However, it can cause serious health issues if left untreated. Regular STI screenings, safe sex practices, and open communication with sexual partners are essential steps in preventing and managing this infection. If you experience any symptoms or believe you may have been exposed to gonorrhea, it is important to seek medical evaluation promptly.

Syphilis

(Caused by Treponema pallidum)

Syphilis is a sexually transmitted infection (STI) caused by the bacterium Treponema pallidum. It is known for its distinct stages and its ability to mimic other diseases, which has historically earned it the nickname "The Great Imitator."

Understanding Syphilis

Syphilis is a bacterial infection usually spread by sexual contact. The disease has several stages, including primary, secondary, latent, and tertiary syphilis, each with different signs and symptoms.

Transmission

Syphilis is primarily spread through:

- Direct contact with a syphilis sore during vaginal, anal, or oral sex.
- It can also be transmitted from an infected mother to her unborn child, known as congenital syphilis.

Symptoms of Syphilis

Primary Syphilis

- Appearance of a single sore (chancre) at the infection site, which is usually firm, round, and painless.
- The sore appears at the location where syphilis entered the body, typically three weeks after exposure.

Secondary Syphilis

- Skin rashes, often on the palms of the hands and soles of the feet.
- Mucous membrane lesions.
- Fever, swollen lymph nodes, sore throat, and fatigue.

Latent Syphilis

- No symptoms are present.
- Can last for years and may progress to tertiary syphilis.

Tertiary Syphilis

- Occurs in a minority of untreated cases.
- Can affect multiple organ systems including the brain, nerves, eyes, heart, blood vessels, liver, bones, and joints.

Congenital Syphilis

- Occurs when syphilis is passed from mother to baby during pregnancy.
- Can lead to miscarriage, stillbirth, or severe health problems in the infant.

Diagnosis of Syphilis

Blood Tests: Commonly used to diagnose syphilis.
Physical Examination: Inspection of any rash or sore.
Cerebrospinal Fluid Test: In cases of neurological involvement.

Treatment for Syphilis

- Penicillin is the standard treatment for all stages of syphilis.
- For those allergic to penicillin, alternative antibiotics are available.

Follow-Up

- Regular blood tests and exams to ensure that the infection is fully cured.
- Sexual partners should also be notified, tested, and treated if necessary.

Prevention of Syphilis

- Using condoms correctly every time you have sex.
- Limiting the number of sexual partners.

- Regular STI screenings, particularly for those with multiple sexual partners or men who have sex with men.

Pregnancy

- All pregnant women should be tested for syphilis early in pregnancy to prevent congenital syphilis.

Syphilis is a serious infection that can cause long-term complications if not treated properly. Early detection and treatment are crucial. Understanding the stages of syphilis and practicing safe sex can greatly reduce the risk of infection. Regular screenings for STIs and open communication with healthcare providers and partners are vital for maintaining sexual health. If you suspect you have been exposed to syphilis, seek medical attention promptly for testing and treatment.

Chancroid

(Caused by Haemophilus ducreyi)

Chancroid is a sexually transmitted infection (STI) caused by the bacterium Haemophilus ducreyi. It is characterized by painful genital ulcers and swollen lymph nodes in the groin area.

Understanding Chancroid

Chancroid is an STI known for causing painful ulcers on the genitalia. It's more common in tropical and subtropical countries and often associated with commercial sex work and drug use.

Transmission

Chancroid is transmitted through sexual contact with an infected person. The bacterium enters the skin during sexual activity, leading to the development of ulcers.

Early Symptoms

- Appearance of small, red bumps on the genitals, which develop into ulcers within a day.
- These ulcers are typically painful, soft, and may bleed easily.

Advanced Symptoms

Enlarged and painful lymph nodes in the groin, which may become abscessed and rupture.

Additional Considerations

- Symptoms usually develop within 4-7 days after exposure.
- The presence of chancroid ulcers can increase the risk of HIV transmission.

Clinical Evaluation

- Examination of genital sores and swollen lymph nodes.
- Consideration of sexual history and potential exposure to STIs.

Laboratory Tests

- Bacterial culture of the ulcer material to detect Haemophilus ducreyi.
- PCR (Polymerase Chain Reaction) tests may also be used, although they are less commonly available.

Treatment for Chancroid

Chancroid is treated with antibiotics such as:

- Azithromycin

- Ceftriaxone
- Erythromycin
- Ciprofloxacin
- Pain Management
- Pain associated with chancroid ulcers can be managed with over-the-counter pain relievers and proper wound care.

Follow-Up

Follow-up visits are necessary to ensure the ulcers are healing and the infection is resolved.

Sexual partners should be examined and treated if they had sexual contact with the patient during the 10 days preceding the patient's onset of symptoms.

Prevention of Chancroid

Use of condoms can reduce the risk of chancroid, although it may not completely prevent the infection due to the possible presence of ulcers outside the covered area.

Limiting the number of sexual partners and avoiding sexual contact with individuals who have genital sores.

Regular Health Check-Ups

Regular screenings for STIs, especially if engaging in high-risk sexual behaviors.

Education and Awareness

Being informed about STIs and their prevention. Open communication with sexual partners about STI risks and testing.

Chancroid is a treatable STI, but it requires prompt medical attention to prevent complications and further spread of the infection. Practicing safe sex, getting regular health check-ups, and being open about sexual health with partners are key steps in managing and preventing chancroid. If you develop painful genital ulcers or swollen lymph nodes in the groin, seek medical care immediately for evaluation and treatment.

Granuloma inguinale

(Caused by Klebsiella granulomatis, formerly known as Calymmatobacterium granulomatis)

Granuloma inguinale, also known as Donovanosis, is a rare sexually transmitted infection (STI) caused by the bacterium Klebsiella granulomatis, formerly known as Calymmatobacterium granulomatis.

Understanding Granuloma Inguinale

Granuloma inguinale is a bacterial infection that leads to the formation of granulomatous ulcers on the genitalia and occasionally in the pelvic region. It is most commonly found in tropical and developing regions.

Transmission

This STI is primarily transmitted through sexual contact. The infection is spread through direct contact with the bacterial lesions of an infected person.

Early Symptoms

- Painless nodules on the genitals or perineal area which may develop into ulcers.
- The ulcers are usually beefy red and bleed easily on contact.

Advanced Symptoms

- The ulcers can grow and cause tissue destruction if not treated.
- In rare cases, the infection can spread to other areas of the body, including the pelvic region, liver, and bones.

Additional Considerations

Symptoms usually develop within one to twelve weeks after exposure.
The ulcers can increase the risk of HIV transmission.

Clinical Examination

- Physical examination of the ulcers.
- Consideration of the patient's sexual history and regions of residence or travel.

Laboratory Tests

- Biopsy of the ulcer to observe Donovan bodies in the tissue, a hallmark of this infection.
- Tissue culture, though it is less commonly used due to the difficulty in culturing the bacteria.

Treatment for Granuloma Inguinale

Antibiotic Therapy

Effective treatment usually involves antibiotics such as:

- Azithromycin
- Doxycycline
- Trimethoprim-sulfamethoxazole
- Erythromycin

Duration of Treatment

Treatment is continued until the ulcers have completely healed, which may take several weeks to months.
Longer treatment duration may be required for advanced cases.

Follow-Up

Regular monitoring of the healing process is necessary.

Sexual partners should be examined and treated if they had contact with the patient within 60 days before the onset of the patient's symptoms.

Prevention of Granuloma Inguinale

Using condoms during sexual activity can reduce the risk of transmission, though they may not completely prevent it.

Limiting the number of sexual partners and avoiding sexual contact with individuals who have genital ulcers.

Regular Health Screenings

- Regular screenings for STIs, particularly for individuals living in or traveling to endemic areas.
- Education and Awareness
- Increasing awareness about STIs and their prevention methods.
- Open communication with sexual partners about sexual health and STI testing.

Granuloma inguinale is a treatable yet potentially severe STI that requires prompt medical intervention. Practicing safe sex, getting regular health check-ups, and maintaining open communication about sexual health with partners are crucial steps in managing and preventing this infection. If you notice any unusual ulcers or lesions in the genital area, it's important to seek medical attention immediately for proper diagnosis and treatment.

Lymphogranuloma venereum

(Caused by Chlamydia trachomatis)

Lymphogranuloma venereum (LGV) is a sexually transmitted infection (STI) caused by specific strains of the bacterium Chlamydia trachomatis. It is characterized by an initial genital lesion followed by swelling and inflammation of the lymphatic tissues.

Understanding Lymphogranuloma Venereum

LGV is an STI caused by three different serovars (types) of Chlamydia trachomatis. It is more invasive than the common chlamydial infection, often leading to significant complications if left untreated.

Transmission

LGV is primarily transmitted through:

- Unprotected vaginal, anal, or oral sex.
- Direct contact with the lesions of an infected person.
- Symptoms of Lymphogranuloma Venereum

Primary Stage

- A small, painless sore or ulcer at the site of infection (usually on the genitals, rectum, or mouth).
- The sore often goes unnoticed and heals within a few days.

Secondary Stage

- Swollen and painful lymph nodes, typically in the groin (buboes).
- Flu-like symptoms, such as fever, muscle aches, and fatigue.
- In rectal infections, symptoms can include rectal pain, discharge, and bleeding.

Tertiary Stage (If Left Untreated)

Chronic inflammation leading to the formation of fistulas and strictures.
Enlargement of the genitalia and swelling of the skin.
Rectal strictures in cases of rectal LGV.
Diagnosis of Lymphogranuloma Venereum

Testing

- Nucleic acid amplification tests (NAATs) to detect Chlamydia trachomatis.
- Specialized testing to differentiate LGV from other chlamydial infections.
- Examination of swollen lymph nodes.

Treatment for Lymphogranuloma Venereum

LGV is treated with a longer course of antibiotics than standard chlamydia infections, such as:

Doxycycline

Erythromycin or azithromycin for those allergic to doxycycline.

Management of Symptoms

- Pain management for swollen lymph nodes.
- Surgical intervention in severe cases with buboes or rectal strictures.

Follow-Up

-
- Follow-up testing to ensure the infection has been cleared.
- Informing and treating sexual partners to prevent reinfection and further spread.

Prevention of Lymphogranuloma Venereum

- Consistent and correct use of condoms during sexual activity.
- Reducing the number of sexual partners.
- Regular STI screenings, particularly for those with multiple partners or men who have sex with men (MSM).

Awareness and Education

Understanding the symptoms and transmission of LGV. Open discussions with healthcare providers and sexual partners about sexual health and STI risks.

Lymphogranuloma venereum is a serious infection that requires prompt and proper treatment to prevent severe complications. Understanding its symptoms and stages, practicing safe sex, and undergoing regular health check-ups are key to managing and preventing LGV. If you experience symptoms such as genital lesions, swollen lymph nodes, or rectal pain, seek medical attention promptly for diagnosis and treatment.

Viral STIs

Human Immunodeficiency Virus

(HIV)/Acquired Immunodeficiency Syndrome (AIDS)

Human Immunodeficiency Virus (HIV) is a virus that attacks the immune system, and if left untreated, it can lead to Acquired Immunodeficiency Syndrome (AIDS), a chronic, potentially life-threatening condition.

Understanding HIV/AIDS

HIV is a virus that targets the immune system, specifically the CD4 cells (T cells), which help the immune system fight off infections. Untreated, HIV reduces the number of CD4 cells, making the person more likely to get infections or infection-related cancers.

Over time, HIV can destroy so many of these cells that the body can't fight off infections and diseases, leading to the most severe phase of the HIV infection, known as AIDS.

Transmission

HIV is transmitted through body fluids that include:

- Blood
- Semen
- Vaginal and rectal fluids
- Breast milk

The virus is spread mainly by:

- Unprotected sexual intercourse with an infected person.
- Sharing needles, syringes, or other items used for injection drug use.
- From mother to child during pregnancy, childbirth, or breastfeeding.

Early Stage of HIV (Acute HIV Infection)

- Flu-like symptoms within 2-4 weeks after the virus enters the body.
- Fever, chills, rash, night sweats, muscle aches, sore throat, fatigue, swollen lymph nodes, mouth ulcers.

Clinical Latency Stage (HIV Inactivity or Dormancy)

- HIV remains in the body and in white blood cells.
- This period is asymptomatic or very mild symptoms.
- Without treatment, this stage lasts about 10 years, but it can last longer.

AIDS (Advanced HIV Infection)

- The most severe phase of HIV infection.
- Rapidly declining immune function.

- Susceptibility to opportunistic infections and cancers.

Diagnosis of HIV/AIDS

Antibody/Antigen Tests: Most commonly used; can detect HIV antibodies and antigens in the blood.

Antibody-Only Tests: Detect HIV antibodies in blood or saliva.

Nucleic Acid Tests (NATs): Look for the actual virus in the blood.

Antiretroviral Therapy (ART)

- Everyone diagnosed with HIV should start ART immediately.
- ART involves taking a combination of HIV medicines every day.
- ART can't cure HIV, but it helps people with HIV live longer, healthier lives.

Managing Side Effects and Coinfections

- Regular monitoring for potential side effects of ART.
- Preventing and treating opportunistic infections.

Prevention of HIV/AIDS

- Consistent use of condoms during sexual intercourse.
- Pre-exposure prophylaxis (PrEP) for people at high risk.
- Post-exposure prophylaxis (PEP) if a recent potential exposure to HIV has occurred.
- Safe needle practices, including using sterile needles and syringes.

Regular Testing

Regular HIV testing, especially for those with risk factors or multiple sexual partners.

Education and Awareness

- Understanding how HIV is transmitted and how to protect yourself.
- Open discussions about HIV status with sexual partners.

HIV/AIDS is a serious health issue, but with early diagnosis and effective treatment, individuals with HIV can live long and healthy lives. Preventive measures, regular testing, and treatment adherence are crucial. It's important to dispel myths and stigmas surrounding HIV/AIDS to encourage awareness, testing, and treatment. If you think you may have been exposed to HIV or are experiencing symptoms, seek medical attention for testing and possible treatment.

Herpes Simplex Virus (HSV) Type 1 and Type 2

The Herpes Simplex Virus (HSV) is a common viral infection that manifests in two types: HSV-1 and HSV-2. Both types can cause sores and blisters around the mouth, genital area, or on other parts of the skin.

Understanding Herpes Simplex Virus

HSV is a virus that causes herpes, which presents as sores or blisters. There are two types:

- HSV-1: Typically causes oral herpes, which is responsible for cold sores around the mouth.
- HSV-2: Usually causes genital herpes.
- Transmission

HSV-1: Spread through oral secretions or sores on the skin, often through kissing, or sharing objects like toothbrushes or eating utensils.

HSV-2: Primarily transmitted through sexual contact with an infected person.

Symptoms of HSV1

- Cold sores or fever blisters on or around the mouth.

- Can also cause genital herpes through oral-genital contact.

Symptoms of HSV-2

- Blisters or sores in the genital area.
- Pain, itching, and small sores followed by scabs in the genital area.

Common Symptoms for Both Types

Pain and discomfort in the affected area.
Itching or burning sensation around the mouth or genitals.
Flu-like symptoms, including fever and swollen lymph nodes, particularly during the first outbreak.

Physical Examination

- Examination of the sores.
- Assessment of symptoms and medical history.

Laboratory Tests

- Viral cultures of the sore.
- Polymerase chain reaction (PCR) tests.
- Blood tests that detect antibodies to HSV-1 or HSV-2.

Antiviral Medications

- Medications such as acyclovir, famciclovir, and valacyclovir.
- These can help to reduce the severity and frequency of symptoms but cannot cure the virus.

Symptom Management

- Pain relievers like ibuprofen or acetaminophen.
- Warm baths and gentle cleansing of the sores.

Managing Recurrences

Antiviral medications can be taken daily to reduce the likelihood of recurrences.
Recognizing and avoiding triggers, such as stress or sun exposure for oral herpes.

Prevention of HSV

- Avoid direct contact with herpes sores.
- Do not share personal items that might have come in contact with the virus.
- Use barrier protection methods, such as condoms, during sexual activities.

Preventing HSV-1 Transmission

- Avoid kissing and oral contact when cold sores are present.

- Avoid sharing items that come in contact with the mouth during an outbreak.

Preventing HSV-2 Transmission

Use condoms or dental dams during sexual contact.
Discuss HSV status with sexual partners.
Consider daily antiviral medication if you have frequent outbreaks or a sexually active partner who is uninfected.

Herpes Simplex Virus, both HSV-1 and HSV-2, are common and manageable conditions. While there is no cure, treatment focuses on managing symptoms and reducing the risk of transmission. Understanding the nature of the virus, practicing safe hygiene and sexual activities, and having open conversations about health status with partners are crucial for managing and preventing HSV. If you suspect you have symptoms of HSV or have been exposed to the virus, seek medical advice for diagnosis and treatment options.

Human Papillomavirus

(HPV) (leading to warts and cervical cancer)

Human Papillomavirus (HPV) is a group of more than 200 related viruses, with more than 40 types transmitted through sexual contact. Some types of HPV can lead to genital warts or certain types of cancer, including cervical cancer.

Understanding Human Papillomavirus (HPV)

HPV is the most common sexually transmitted infection (STI). While most HPV infections go away on their own without causing any health problems, some can cause genital warts, and others can lead to cancers in different parts of the body, including the cervix, oropharynx, anus, rectum, penis, vagina, and vulva.

Types of HPV

- Low-risk HPVs: Typically cause warts, including genital warts.
- High-risk HPVs: Can lead to cancer.

Transmission of HPV

- Sexual and Skin-to-Skin Contact
- HPV is transmitted primarily through intimate skin-to-skin contact, not just penetrative sex.

- Genital warts are spread through sexual contact.
- You can get HPV even if you have sex with a person who has no signs or symptoms.

Symptoms of HPV

Genital Warts
- Small or large, raised or flat, or cauliflower-shaped warts on the genital area.
- May appear weeks or months after sexual contact with an infected person.

Cancer Symptoms

- HPV-related cancers often don't have symptoms until they are quite advanced and hard to treat.
- Regular screenings for cervical cancer (Pap test and HPV test) are essential for women.

Visual Examination

Diagnosis of genital warts is usually made by visual inspection.

Pap Test and HPV Test

- Pap test (or Pap smear) checks for cell changes on the cervix that might become cervical cancer if left untreated.
- HPV test looks for the virus that can cause these cell changes.

Treatment for Warts

- Treatments include topical medications, cryotherapy, surgical removal, and laser therapy.
- Over-the-counter treatments for non-genital warts should not be used for genital warts.

Management of Cancer-Causing HPV

- Regular cervical screening to detect precancerous changes, which can be treated before they turn into cancer.
- Treatment for cancers caused by HPV depends on the type, location, and stage of the cancer.

Prevention of HPV

HPV Vaccine

Vaccination is available and recommended for boys and girls to protect against the types of HPV that most commonly cause cancer and genital warts.

Safe Sex Practices

Condoms can lower the risk of contracting HPV, but they do not provide complete protection because HPV can infect areas not covered by a condom.

Regular Health Check-Ups

- Regular cervical screening for women.
- Awareness of changes in the body and seeking medical advice if you notice anything unusual.

HPV is a common virus, with certain types posing significant health risks, including the development of genital warts and various cancers. Vaccination, safe sex practices, and regular health screenings are key in managing and preventing HPV infections. If you suspect you have been exposed to HPV, or if you have symptoms of genital warts or other related health issues, consult with a healthcare provider for appropriate testing and treatment.

Hepatitis B

(and less commonly Hepatitis A and C, which can be transmitted sexually under certain circumstances)

Hepatitis is an inflammation of the liver, commonly caused by a viral infection.

Understanding Hepatitis B

Hepatitis B is a liver infection caused by the Hepatitis B virus (HBV). It can range in severity from a mild illness lasting a few weeks to a serious, lifelong illness.

Transmission of Hepatitis B

- Sexual contact with an infected person.
- Sharing needles, syringes, or other drug-injection equipment.
- From mother to baby at birth.
- Contact with the blood or open sores of an infected person.

Symptoms of Hepatitis B

- Yellowing of the skin and eyes (jaundice).
- Pain and swelling in the abdomen.
- Dark urine and pale-colored stool.
- Chronic fatigue.
- Fever and flu-like symptoms.

Diagnosis and Treatment of Hepatitis B

Blood tests to detect the presence of HBV antigens and antibodies.

Treatment

- Acute Hepatitis B usually requires no specific treatment.
- Chronic Hepatitis B is treated with antiviral medications to reduce liver damage.
- Regular monitoring for liver function and possible liver damage is crucial.

Hepatitis A

- Usually spreads through ingestion of contaminated food or water.
- Sexual transmission can occur, particularly among men who have sex with men (MSM).
- Vaccination is available and effective.

Hepatitis C

- Primarily spread through blood-to-blood contact.
- Less commonly, it can be transmitted sexually, especially among individuals with HIV, MSM, and those who engage in high-risk sexual behaviors.
- Chronic Hepatitis C is treated with antiviral medications.

Symptoms of Hepatitis A and C

- Both can cause jaundice, fatigue, abdominal pain, loss of appetite, and nausea.
- Symptoms of Hepatitis C might not appear for many years until significant liver damage has occurred.

Vaccination

- Hepatitis B and A vaccines provide effective immunity.
- There is no vaccine for Hepatitis C.

Safe Practices

- Using condoms during sexual activity.
- Avoiding sharing needles and personal items like razors or toothbrushes.
- Screening and vaccination for individuals at risk.

Hepatitis B is a significant health concern, particularly due to its mode of transmission and potential chronicity. Hepatitis A and C, while less commonly sexually transmitted, also pose health risks. Prevention through vaccination, safe sex practices, and regular health check-ups are key to managing and mitigating the risks associated with these diseases. If you believe you have been exposed to any form of hepatitis or exhibit symptoms, it's important to get tested and seek medical care promptly.

Molluscum contagiosum

(virus causing skin lesions)

Molluscum contagiosum is a viral skin infection that causes raised, pearl-like papules or nodules on the skin. It's caused by the molluscum contagiosum virus (MCV), a member of the poxvirus family.

Understanding Molluscum Contagiosum

Molluscum contagiosum is a common, contagious skin infection that typically affects children, but can also occur in adults, particularly those with weakened immune systems or through sexual contact.

Transmission

- Direct skin-to-skin contact.
- Contact with contaminated objects, such as towels or clothing.
- In adults, it can be sexually transmitted.

Symptoms of Molluscum Contagiosum

Small, firm, raised spots on the skin, typically pearl-like and flesh-colored.

Lesions can appear anywhere on the body, but are most common on the face, arms, and legs in children, and the genitals, lower abdomen, and inner thigh in adults.

The spots are usually painless but can become itchy, sore, red, and swollen.

Clinical Examination

- Diagnosis is usually made based on the appearance of the lesions.
- A dermatologist can typically diagnose molluscum contagiosum by examining the affected skin.

Biopsy

In uncertain cases, a biopsy of the lesion may be performed for a definitive diagnosis.

Treatment Options

In many cases, particularly in children, treatment may not be necessary as the condition usually resolves on its own within 6 to 12 months.

- Cryotherapy (freezing off the lesions).
- Curettage (surgical removal of the lesions).
- Topical treatments (chemicals to induce blistering and removal of the lesions).

- Laser therapy.

Home Care

- Avoid scratching or picking at the lesions to prevent spreading the virus to other parts of the body or to other people.
- Keep the affected area clean and covered.

Preventive Measures

- Avoid sharing personal items like towels, clothing, and razors.
- Practice good personal hygiene.
- In adults, using condoms can reduce the risk of sexual transmission, but it may not prevent skin-to-skin transmission completely.

In Children

Teach children about the importance of handwashing and not sharing personal items.
Keep children with molluscum contagiosum out of swimming pools, if possible, to prevent spreading the virus.

Molluscum contagiosum is a common viral infection that results in distinctive skin lesions. It's generally harmless and resolves on its own, but treatment can be sought for cosmetic reasons or if the lesions are bothersome. Understanding how the virus spreads and taking appropriate preventive measures can help reduce the risk of infection or transmission. If you or your child has symptoms of molluscum contagiosum, consult a healthcare provider for proper diagnosis and advice on management options.

Parasitic STIs

Trichomoniasis

(caused by Trichomonas vaginalis)

Trichomoniasis is a common sexually transmitted infection (STI) caused by the parasite Trichomonas vaginalis. It can affect both men and women, but symptoms are more common in women.

Understanding Trichomoniasis

Trichomoniasis, often referred to as "trich," is an STI caused by the protozoan parasite Trichomonas vaginalis. The infection affects the urogenital tract, primarily the vagina in women and the urethra in men.

Transmission

Trichomoniasis is mainly transmitted through sexual intercourse.
The parasite is usually spread from penis to vagina or from vagina to vagina. It is less commonly transmitted to other body parts.

Symptoms In Women

- Vaginal discharge that is often yellow-green, frothy, and has an unpleasant smell.
- Pain during urination or sexual intercourse.
- Itching or irritation inside the vagina.

- Lower abdominal discomfort (less common).

Symptoms In Men

- Discharge from the penis.
- Burning sensation after urination or ejaculation.
- Itching or irritation inside the penis.

Asymptomatic Cases

- Many people with trichomoniasis do not develop any symptoms.
- Asymptomatic individuals can still transmit the infection to others.

Diagnosis of Trichomoniasis

Physical examination: A healthcare provider may notice signs of the infection during a pelvic examination.

Laboratory tests: The most definitive way to diagnose trichomoniasis is through laboratory tests, which can include a microscopic examination of the discharge, a rapid antigen test, or a nucleic acid amplification test (NAAT).

Treatment for Trichomoniasis

- Trichomoniasis is generally treated with a single dose of an antibiotic, usually metronidazole or tinidazole.

- It's important for all sexual partners to be treated at the same time to prevent reinfection.

During Treatment

Avoid alcohol consumption during treatment and for 24 hours after taking metronidazole or 72 hours after taking tinidazole, as mixing the drug with alcohol can cause severe nausea and vomiting.

Prevention of Trichomoniasis

- Using condoms correctly every time during sexual intercourse significantly reduces the risk of contracting trichomoniasis.
- Limiting the number of sexual partners.

Regular Testing

Routine STI screening, especially for sexually active individuals with multiple partners.

Avoiding Douching

Women should avoid douching as it can disrupt the natural balance of bacteria and yeasts in the vagina, increasing the risk of infections.

Trichomoniasis is a treatable STI, but it requires prompt attention to prevent complications and the spread of the infection. Practicing safe sex, undergoing regular STI screenings, and seeking timely treatment are essential for managing trichomoniasis. If you experience symptoms suggestive of trichomoniasis or have been sexually active with multiple partners, it is advisable to get tested and seek appropriate treatment.

Pubic lice

("crabs," caused by Pthirus pubis)

Pubic lice, commonly known as "crabs," are tiny parasitic insects that infest the hair in the pubic region. Caused by Pthirus pubis, they are a common sexually transmitted infestation.

Understanding Pubic Lice

Pubic lice are small lice that infest the coarse hair of the genital area. They can also be found in other coarse body hair, such as hair on the legs, armpits, mustache, beard, eyebrows, and eyelashes.

Transmission

- Pubic lice are most commonly transmitted through sexual contact.
- They can also be spread through contact with infested clothing, bedding, or towels.

Symptoms of Pubic Lice

- Itching in the affected area, which is usually more intense at night.
- Blue spots or small specks of blood on the skin, which are lice excrement.

- Visible nits (lice eggs) or crawling lice in the pubic hair.
- Mild fever and feeling run-down (less common).

Visual Inspection

- The diagnosis is typically made by visually identifying the lice or nits in the pubic hair.
- A magnifying glass may be used to help see the lice or nits.

Over-the-Counter Lotions and Shampoos

- Permethrin lotion or pyrethrin with piperonyl butoxide can be used to treat the infestation.
- Follow the instructions on the medication label carefully.

Prescription Medications

If over-the-counter treatments don't work, your healthcare provider may prescribe stronger medication.

Additional Measures

Wash clothing, bedding, and towels used in the two days before treatment in hot water and dry them on a hot setting.

Items that can't be washed may be sealed in a plastic bag for two weeks.

Avoid sexual contact until you and your partner(s) have completed treatment and no longer have symptoms.

Treating Close Contacts

Sexual partners and other close contacts should be treated at the same time to prevent re-infestation.

Prevention of Pubic Lice
-
- Limiting the number of sexual partners.
- Using condoms may help reduce the risk but does not fully prevent the spread of pubic lice.

Personal Hygiene and Care

Avoid sharing clothing, bedding, and towels with others. Regular washing of clothing and bedding in hot water.

Pubic lice are a common and treatable condition. It's important to follow proper treatment procedures and take steps to avoid re-infestation. Maintaining good personal hygiene and being cautious about sharing personal items can help prevent the spread of pubic lice. If you suspect you have pubic lice, it's advisable to seek treatment promptly and inform any recent sexual partners so they can also be treated if necessary.

Scabies

(caused by the mite Sarcoptes scabiei)

Scabies is a contagious skin condition caused by the mite Sarcoptes scabiei. These tiny mites burrow into the skin, causing itching and rash.

Understanding Scabies

Scabies is an infestation of the skin by the human itch mite Sarcoptes scabiei var. hominis. The mites burrow into the top layer of skin where they live and lay eggs.

Transmission

Scabies is spread through:

- Prolonged direct skin-to-skin contact with an infected person.
- Less commonly, scabies can be spread by sharing clothing, towels, or bedding with someone who has an infestation.

Symptoms of Scabies

- Intense itching, especially at night.
- A pimple-like rash.
- Scales or blisters.
- Sores caused by scratching.

The most common areas affected are the webs between fingers, wrists, elbows, armpits, waist, buttocks, and genital area.

Physical Examination

A healthcare provider will examine the skin for signs of scabies.

Skin Scraping

In some cases, a doctor may perform a skin scraping to look for mites, eggs, or mite fecal matter under a microscope.

Topical Scabicides

- Prescription creams and lotions are applied all over the body, usually from the neck down, and left on for a prescribed period before washing off.
- Permethrin cream 5% is the most commonly prescribed medication for treating scabies.

Oral Medications

In some cases, oral medications like ivermectin may be prescribed.

Treating All Contacts

It's important to treat all family members and close contacts, even if they don't have symptoms.

After Treatment

Itching may continue for several weeks, but this does not mean the treatment was ineffective.

Prevention of Scabies

Avoid Direct Contact

Avoid prolonged skin-to-skin contact with someone who has scabies.

Personal Items

Do not share clothing, bedding, or towels with someone who has scabies.

Clean and Disinfect

- Wash all clothing, towels, and bedding used by the infested person in hot water and dry in a hot dryer.
- Vacuum furniture and carpets where the infested person sat or lay.

Scabies is a highly contagious skin condition but is treatable with prescription medication. Prompt treatment for you and your close contacts, as well as thorough cleaning and disinfection of your environment, are important steps in managing a scabies infestation. If you suspect you have scabies, consult with a healthcare provider for diagnosis and treatment. Remember, continued itching for a few weeks after treatment does not necessarily mean the scabies mites are still present.

Other STIs

Bacterial Vaginosis

(caused by various types of bacteria, not always transmitted sexually but associated with sexual activity)

Bacterial Vaginosis (BV) is a common vaginal condition caused by an imbalance in the natural bacteria in the vagina. While not always transmitted sexually, it is associated with sexual activity.

Understanding Bacterial Vaginosis

Bacterial Vaginosis is the most common vaginal infection in women of childbearing age. It occurs when the normal balance of bacteria in the vagina is disrupted and replaced by an overgrowth of certain bacteria.

Causes

- The exact cause of BV is not fully understood.
- It's associated with having multiple sexual partners, a new sexual partner, or douching.
- BV is not considered an STI, but it can develop after sexual intercourse with a new partner.

Symptoms of Bacterial Vaginosis

- Thin, gray, white or green vaginal discharge.
- A fishy odor, especially after sex.
- Burning during urination.

- Itching around the outside of the vagina.

Asymptomatic Cases

Many women with BV have no symptoms and only discover the condition through a pelvic examination.

Pelvic Examination

A healthcare provider may notice signs of BV during a pelvic exam.

Laboratory Tests

- Testing the pH level of the vaginal fluid.
- Looking at a sample of vaginal discharge under a microscope.
- Bacterial culture is not typically needed for diagnosis.

Treatment for Bacterial Vaginosis

- BV is typically treated with antibiotic medication, either oral or vaginal.
- Common antibiotics include metronidazole, clindamycin, and tinidazole.

Follow-up

- Symptoms usually improve within a few days after starting the antibiotic.

- It's important to complete the entire course of antibiotics, even if symptoms go away.

Recurrent BV

Women who have recurrent BV may need longer treatment or a maintenance plan.

Prevention of Bacterial Vaginosis

- Limiting the number of sexual partners.
- Avoiding douching as it disrupts the natural balance of bacteria in the vagina.
- Using condoms may help to prevent BV.

Lifestyle Changes

- Probiotics may help to maintain the natural balance of bacteria in the vagina.
- Regular gynecological check-ups.

Bacterial Vaginosis is a common condition that results from an imbalance in the natural bacteria in the vagina. While it can be associated with sexual activity, it is not strictly an STI. BV is treatable with antibiotics, and women experiencing symptoms should consult their healthcare provider for diagnosis and treatment. Maintaining a healthy vaginal environment and practicing safe sexual practices are key to preventing BV. If you suspect you have BV or are experiencing symptoms, it is important to seek medical attention for proper diagnosis and treatment.

Mycoplasma genitalium infection

Mycoplasma genitalium (M. genitalium) is a sexually transmitted bacterium that can cause urogenital infections. While it was identified in the 1980s, its significance as a sexually transmitted infection (STI) has only recently been recognized.

Understanding Mycoplasma Genitalium

Mycoplasma genitalium is a small bacterium that infects the mucosal surfaces of the urogenital tract. It's increasingly recognized as a cause of urethritis in men and has been associated with several conditions in women, including cervicitis and pelvic inflammatory disease.

Transmission

- The primary mode of transmission is through sexual contact.
- It can be transmitted through vaginal, anal, or possibly oral sex.
- Symptoms of Mycoplasma Genitalium

In Men

- Urethritis, which can cause pain or burning during urination.
- Discharge from the penis.

In Women

- Cervicitis, with symptoms such as vaginal discharge and bleeding after sex or between periods.
- Pelvic inflammatory disease (PID), with symptoms including pelvic pain, fever, and general discomfort.

Asymptomatic Cases

Many individuals infected with Mycoplasma genitalium do not show symptoms but can still transmit the infection to others.

Testing

Nucleic acid amplification tests (NAATs) are used to detect M. genitalium in urine samples or genital swabs. These tests are not widely available in all healthcare settings.

Treatment for Mycoplasma Genitalium

- Antibiotic treatment is the primary method for treating M. genitalium infections.
- Azithromycin is commonly used, but resistance to this antibiotic is increasing.
- Alternatives like moxifloxacin may be considered, especially in cases of treatment failure.

Treatment Challenges

- Emerging antibiotic resistance makes treatment challenging.
- Repeat testing post-treatment is recommended to ensure the infection has been cleared.

Prevention of Mycoplasma Genitalium

- Consistent and correct use of condoms during sexual intercourse to reduce the risk of transmission.
- Limiting the number of sexual partners.

Regular STI Screening

Regular screening for STIs, especially for individuals with new or multiple sexual partners.

Awareness and Communication

- Being aware of the signs and symptoms of STIs.
- Open communication with sexual partners about STIs and STI testing.

Mycoplasma genitalium is a relatively new addition to the list of STIs and poses unique challenges due to its emerging antibiotic resistance. Understanding its transmission, symptoms, and the importance of safe sex practices is crucial for its prevention and control. If you experience symptoms suggestive of a urogenital infection or have multiple sexual partners, consider getting tested for M. genitalium and other STIs. Early diagnosis and appropriate treatment are key to managing this infection effectively.

Ureaplasma urealyticum infection

Ureaplasma urealyticum is a type of bacteria that is commonly found in the human urogenital tract. While it is often present without causing symptoms, it can sometimes lead to infections, particularly in the urinary and reproductive systems.

Understanding Ureaplasma Urealyticum

Ureaplasma urealyticum is part of the normal genital flora in many individuals but can cause disease in certain situations. It's a small bacterium unenclosed by a cell wall, which makes it unique among bacteria and affects the types of antibiotics that can be used against it.

Transmission

- Sexual contact is the most common method of transmission.
- It can also be transmitted from mother to baby during childbirth.

Symptoms In Men

Non-gonococcal urethritis (inflammation of the urethra not caused by gonorrhea), presenting with symptoms like burning during urination and discharge from the penis.

Symptoms In Women

- Urethritis, cervicitis, and pelvic inflammatory disease (PID), with symptoms such as vaginal discharge, pelvic pain, and pain during intercourse.
- It may also be associated with infertility.

Asymptomatic Cases

Many people infected with Ureaplasma urealyticum do not show any symptoms but can still transmit the bacterium to others.

Laboratory Testing

Nucleic acid amplification tests (NAATs) from urine samples or genital swabs are used to detect the presence of Ureaplasma urealyticum.

Culture methods can also be used but are less common.

Treatment for Ureaplasma Urealyticum Infection

- Tetracycline antibiotics like doxycycline are often the first line of treatment.

- Macrolide antibiotics such as azithromycin can be used in case of tetracycline resistance or intolerance.
- Fluoroquinolones are another alternative, especially in complicated cases.

Considerations in Treatment

- Due to the risk of developing antibiotic resistance, accurate diagnosis and appropriate antibiotic selection are crucial.
- Sexual partners should be treated simultaneously to prevent reinfection.

Prevention of Ureaplasma Urealyticum Infection

Using condoms during sexual intercourse can reduce the risk of transmission.
Limiting the number of sexual partners and engaging in mutual monogamy.

Regular STI Screening

Regular screening for STIs is important, especially for those with new or multiple sexual partners.

Awareness and Education

- Understanding the potential risks and symptoms associated with common urogenital infections.

- Open communication with sexual partners about sexual health and STI testing.

Ureaplasma urealyticum is a common bacterium that can lead to various urogenital infections. Being aware of its existence, understanding the symptoms it may cause, and engaging in safe sexual practices are essential for prevention. If you suspect you might have a Ureaplasma infection or are experiencing symptoms of a urogenital infection, seek medical advice for testing and appropriate treatment. Early diagnosis and treatment are key to managing this infection effectively.

Made in the USA
Columbia, SC
05 May 2024

35312928R00043